I0789864

# Five Beliefs That Are Keeping You Fat…
## and how to clear them

TAMARA PITELEN

Copyright © 2017 Tamara Pitelen Awakenings Books

All rights reserved. No part of this booklet may be reproduced by any mechanical, photographic, or electronic process, or in the form of a phonographic recording; nor may it be stored in a retrieval system, transmitted, or otherwise be copied for public or private use—other than for "fair use" as brief quotations embodied in articles and reviews—without prior written permission of the author. To request permission, email tamara@awakeningsuk.com.
The information in this booklet is not intended as a replacement for medical advice nor does it prescribe the use of any technique as a form of treatment for physical, emotional, or medical problems without the advice of a physician, either directly or indirectly. The intent is to offer general information with regards to emotional well-being. In the event you use any of the information in this book for yourself, the author and the publisher assume no responsibility for your actions.

ISBN: 1976272874
ISBN-13: 978-1976272875

# CONTENTS

# INTRODUCTION

Let's get straight to the heart of the matter: if you've been trying
and failing to shed excess body fat for a long time then there's a
part of you that wants that weight.
That's right, that's what I said, some subconscious part of you
*wants* that weight and this part of you has really good reasons.
If there was not a part of you that wanted the extra weight, it
wouldn't be there because you and your body would easily shed
it. I spent decades wasting my life on dieting and exercise before I
realised I needed to reprogram my brain before any changes to
my lifestyle would make any difference. As a result this is what I
now believe in a nutshell...

... your weight problem won't be solved only by focusing on food
and exercise. Dieting does NOT work.

... If you're carrying excess weight, your subconscious mind
wants it as defense against emotional and mental stresses and it
will set off a storm of hormonal havoc and cravings to hold onto
this excess weight

... this mental and emotional stress comes from our past or current
life experiences, as well as from the resulting beliefs and
programming

... this can all be boiled down to the BEEBs: **Beliefs**, **Emotions**, **Events** and **Benefits**.

By working on your BEEBs you will finally release the excess weight effortlessly because your body-mind will be working with you instead of fighting against you.

Before we go any further though, let me tell you a little about my journey. I spent decades jumping every hoop the diet industry threw to try and lose weight. I'll tell you more about that in the coming chapters but here are some of the highlights...

- At age nine, a doctor put me on my first low calorie diet
- Ten years of dieting later, I peaked at my heaviest weight, about 45lbs (20kg) more than I weigh today
- I've spent 30 years on a diet (insane, literally!) - decades of misery-bingeing and crash-dieting along with punishing exercise routines and stress-eating
- I did excessive exercise (I ran marathons and other long distance running, triathlons, aerobics teacher, three months cycling around Ireland...)
- I was trapped in a vicious cycle of self-blame, self-punishment and self-criticism, I put my life on hold, was OBSESSED with my weight, with calories, with what I ate...
- I felt hopeless, I often ended up in tears because it felt like my body was battling with me every step of the way (it was)
- The dieting triggered eating disorders, cravings, binges... which led to metabolic syndrome, insulin resistance, leptin resistance, famine response, low metabolism, thyroid and hormonal disorders, digestive disorders... it was a cascade of knock on issues that led to more weight gain. My body became a frighteningly efficient fat storing machine.

# 1 THE FAT GIRL SINGS

I was aged just nine when a doctor put me on my first low calorie diet.

It was the late 1970s and the billion dollar dieting industry was just starting to get into full swing. We were all buying into the theories about how low calorie diets and low fat Frankenfoods were the answer to weight loss. On the surface, it seemed to make all the sense in the world - just stop eating fat and you'll stop having fat on your body, we thought. But if the past 40 hysterical fat-phobic years have taught us anything it's that such a simplistic view of the human body and metabolism is just stupid.

Fast forward 40 years to today and where has all that calorie counting and zero per cent fat yogurt got us? It's dropkicked us straight into a critical global obesity crisis that's unprecedented in human history.

Let's go back for a moment though to the nine-year-old me though who was walking home with my mum from that doctor's surgery grasping a joyless bit of paper that barked orders like, 'breakfast: half a grapefruit with black tea or coffee'.

This regime allowed me 800 to 1,000 calories a day – which was the accepted wisdom of the time for anyone wanting to reduce weight, no matter whether they were nine or 90 years old.

'Just consume 1,000 calories a day and you will lose weight' the experts told us. 'It's that easy, no arguments. If you can't do it then you're just lazy and not trying hard enough.'

It was the lie we all bought. Today's massively profitable diet industry was built on that premise.

For me, the only thing that decades of deprivation, calorie counting, and punishing exercise regimes did was make me feel like a failure, make me obsessive and miserable. It also triggered a storm of eating disorders, cravings, and binges that led to metabolic syndrome, insulin resistance, leptin resistance, famine response, thyroid and hormonal disorders, sluggish metabolism, digestive disorders, lethargy… it was a cascade of knock-on issues that led to more and more weight gain.

I actually dieted myself fatter and unwell!

At 19 years old, after 10 years of dieting, I peaked at my heaviest weight, which was about 20kgs (45lbs) more than I weigh today because, instead of helping me shift that little bit of excess fat off my nine-year-old body, all that dieting triggered real problems -- physical, mental and emotional. And it ignored the real reasons for the extra weight that had so quickly manifested: reasons that had nothing to do with food and everything to do with love.

## YOUR SUBCONSCIOUS ALWAYS WINS

Let me get straight to the bottom line. If you're carrying excess body fat that just won't budge, or might go away but always comes back, it's because some part of your subconscious brain wants this extra weight.

I'm going to say that again because this is the important bit – part of you WANTS this extra body fat. I know. It's hard to swallow, isn't it (unlike that tub of cookie dough ice-cream).

Consciously, you'd go to all sorts of ridiculous lengths to get rid of this excess body fat – from starving yourself on cabbage juice to buying some machine off the shopping channel at 2am - but subconsciously you have good reasons for keeping it.

Neuroscientists tell us that that the conscious mind accounts for just five per cent of our cognitive activity. That means that about 95 per cent of our decisions, actions, emotions, patterns and behaviours are derived from the processing of the subconscious mind, also called the unconscious mind.

So in a battle between the two minds, the subconscious always wins. It doesn't matter what you consciously want. Your conscious mind has the firepower of a cigarette lighter in comparison to your subconscious mind's fleet of nuclear warships. This is why putting your faith in willpower is a huge waste of time.

Every single behaviour that you demonstrate, good, bad, frightening, or ridiculous, is run by your subconscious mind. So if you want to change a behaviour, you cannot do it by willpower alone, you have to get into the subconscious mind and change it there. That's when transformation takes place.

## RELEASING EMOTIONAL BODY FAT BAGGAGE

So what needs to happen for you to release your excess body fat? The key is in figuring out how the weight is serving you and uprooting the old core beliefs attached to this so that your subconscious mind no longer perceives a benefit in holding onto the excess weight.

Once your subconscious mind no longer wants the weight, it will change all the settings in your body to begin releasing the excess fat. For example, it will raise your metabolism, decrease your appetite and turn off your cravings. It'll start burning fat for fuel instead of muscle, it will start laying down more muscle, and it will activate your satiety messages. And more. Your subconscious mind has all sorts of tools up its sleeves for changing your physicality.

So what kind of beliefs might be hidden in your subconscious mind that are sabotaging your weight-loss efforts? In truth, the possibilities are endless because every one of us is different with a unique set of circumstances and life experiences.

My reasons for holding onto body fat are unique to me and to my life experiences and inherited genetic coding, as your reasons are to you. Having said that, from what I've observed through working with many other people using the ThetaHealing

Technique and EFT Tapping, most of these reasons can be boiled down to five universal core beliefs, which are listed below:

**Fat is love:**
You have wonderful memories of eating food with people who love you and who nurtured you so you turn to food to feel loved and nurtured. Food is how you nurture yourself, how you treat yourself and how you reward yourself. Trouble is, the resulting excess fat is also seen by the body-mind as love and comfort so you hold onto it to feel loved. Similarly, you might have had a grandmother who showered you with love and affection and you have some deep memories of her soft fat belly or her large shelf of a bosom. At some level, your own soft fat belly reminds you of her and that feeling of being completely enveloped in her unconditional love and doting. Of course you're going to want to be reminded of that! And if you can carry this love with you always simply by having a big soft belly, who would blame you? But of course consciously, you don't want that 'unsightly' belly so you deny yourself the foods that comfort you and make you feel loved. When you do this, at some level it feels like abuse from a critical and unloving parental figure, even rejection. So eventually you'll rebel against that 'punishment' and go on a binge-eating session of these foods as both rebellion and for comfort.

**Fat is protection:**
This is when people use body fat to avoid unwanted sexual attention or as a buffer against emotional abuse. Subconsciously, people make themselves unattractive to avoid the wrong kind of attention. Also, the extra weight literally puts more distance between them and the abuser. This can be emotional or mental abuse as well as physical, a bullying boss for example. However, fat as protection can also be about protecting yourself

from heavy metals and toxins. If at some point in your life, or over time, you were exposed to heavy metals such as fluoride, mercury or lead, the body may be protecting your delicate internal organs and brain from these substances by basically locking them away in your fat cells as a kind of quarantine. The solution is a period of cellular detoxification with, say, green juices and spirulina, coupled with working on releasing the beliefs that keep some part of you resonating with the frequency of these toxic substances.

**Fat is safety:**
There are countless ways that excess weight can make us feel safer. For example, some people gain weight when they get married as a way to avoid being unfaithful. Or they feel safer with – literally – some extra weight to back them up and support them. The subconscious belief and benefit could be something like, 'they can't push me around if I'm heavy'.
For some of us, we literally create a suit of armour with body fat. We surround ourselves in fat in so that other people can't get close to us. We believe we are keeping ourselves safe by doing so.
Alternatively, if someone was taught that everyone in their family is overweight and in order to belong in the family they must be overweight as well, then holding onto excess fat allows them to perpetuate this belief and remain in the family unit where they feel safe.

**Fat is an excuse:**
Excess weight is also a great excuse for not doing something we're afraid to do, for example, 'I'll start dating/ travel/ go skydiving / learn to swim / get a new job… when I lose weight.' Why do we procrastinate? Usually out of fear; fear of change, fear of failure, even fear of success – say you succeed in getting

that amazing new job or promotion, will that mean longer hours, harder work, no life-work balance, more competition…? And will that ruin your marriage and impact your health? Or maybe you've picked up beliefs from your parents that 'life is a struggle' and 'nothing worthwhile comes without struggle' so you are subconsciously ensuring that you keep struggling in order to feel worthy (that was one of mine!).

**Fat is survival:**
If someone has financial or job worries, or if their ancestors experienced famine or starvation and the experience is now coded in their DNA, this can result in holding onto excess weight.
In our lizard brain, we know we are more likely to survive the winter or a famine if we have extra fat and in our lizard brain, the 21st century worry about not being able to pay the mortgage is the same as the Neanderthal man's worry about dying of starvation. Solution? Build up the fat stores.
This one can also get complex if you have a hormonal condition such as an underactive thyroid. This can mean that you are leptin resistant so that your brain cannot 'see' all the fat on your body. So even though you're carrying, say, 20 or 200 kilos of excess fat, your brain doesn't 'see' it because the leptin messages aren't getting through to your hypothalamus. So the brain keeps instructing the body's systems to store fat because it actually thinks you're starving. Then, when your brain already thinks you're starving and you then start another low calorie diet and do more exercise, all you're doing is making your brain really panic about your survival and it will then go into overdrive on working even harder to keep the fat where it is. So your brain hits the panic button and puts all your systems on emergency survival mode – cue massive cravings for chocolate, a snail-like metabolism, and muscle burning for fuel instead of fat. Because as far as your brain is concerned, your actions make as much

sense as a person who's starving to death deciding to run a marathon.

These five belief themes incorporate just some of the many good reasons we have for holding onto excess body fat as padding. We also use excess weight to feel grounded, to define our boundaries, to provide a buffer between us and the world.

And here's the other point to make. You will probably have more than one, if not all, of these beliefs all jumbled together, overlapping and interweaving… so your mission, should you choose to accept it, is to go within and go deep. To uncover and uproot the reasons you have for keeping the excess weight. And then, when you finally no longer need it, it'll simply melt away. So, shall we get started, you gorgeous thing?

# 2 HOW TO TAP FOR BEGINNERS

Before we jump into the EFT Tapping scripts, you'll need to know how to actually do EFT Tapping. Don't worry, the basics are very simple. If you already know how to tap, please just jump ahead to the next chapter. If you're new to the world of EFT Tapping, I'll offer an introduction here but there are a myriad of excellent and free resources out there prepared by people far more expert than I am in this modality and I would encourage you to explore the work of these wonderful people – in particular I'd like to acknowledge the people who brought this incredible technique to the world, namely Roger Callahan and Gary Craig. Some excellent places for you to do further and more indepth research are the following websites:

www.emofree.com
www.eft-universe.com
www.TheTappingSolution.com

Here's the brief overview though: EFT Tapping is an amazingly powerful yet simple – and free - healing technique that can have you shifting your life within minutes.
EFT stands for Emotional Freedom Techniques, which is its

proper but more tongue-tying name. The even more user-friendly term for it is Tapping, so called because it involves using your fingertips to tap on specific points on your head and body.

In simple terms, EFT or Tapping is a blend of ancient Chinese medicine and modern western psychology. You can think of it as like acupuncture without the needles and it can free you from persistent or inappropriate negative emotions, in other words, stuck or blocked nervous energy in one or more of your nerve channels, or meridians.

If you think of your energetic system as an energy motorway, then a past trauma is a little like a car crash or traffic jam on that motorway. Something is stopping the energy – or traffic – from flowing and this causes problems that can then manifest into physical issues.

How does EFT Tapping work? In the most simple terms, this light tapping on the endpoints of the primary energy meridians in your body sends a calming signal to the amygdala – which is the brain's alarm bell and the trigger for the fight, freeze or flight response.

Whenever you're in a stressful situation or you simply think of something that causes you stress - and for some people this could be just the thought of standing on the bathroom scales in the morning – then your body responds to this thought by pumping out stress hormones like cortisol and adrenalin, by diverting resources to your extremities and away from your non-essential functions like digestion, by increasing your heart rate and breathing to pull in more oxygen so the muscles can fight or flee. This process also sees the more creative and lateral thinking parts of the brain shut down so you're operating from the primal lizard brain – in other words you actually become more stupid when you're in the stress response and are unable to think of solutions beyond 'run for your life!' or 'fight for your life!'

## 1. Identify the issue

This could be any physical, emotional, mental or spiritual issue. For example, a sore shoulder or anxiety around losing a job. For people wanting to deal with weight, it could be 'I hate my fat belly' or 'I'll never find a soul mate until I lose this weight'. Physically, it could be 'my back aches from all this excess weight'.

## 2. Rate the intensity of pain or distress from 0-10

If it's physical pain, how sore is it on a scale from zero to 10? If it's an emotional challenge, how upset or distressed are you?

## 3. Set-up statement

While tapping with two or three fingers on the fleshy side of either hand, just below the little finger, also called the karate chop point, we just plainly state the issue. For example, 'I've got this chronic back ache' or 'I'm really stressed about money'

We say the set-up statement three times and there are two aims to achieve by doing this. First, you're acknowledging the problem or issue. You're shining the light on it and pulling it out from where it's been hiding in the dark. And, second, you're accepting and loving yourself in spite of it.

So a typical set-up statement would be: "Even though I'm stressed to the max about all the debt I'm in and I can't see a way out of it, I accept that I feel this way and I completely love and forgive myself anyway." (Funnily enough, weight and abundance issues are very often connected at a subconscious level – for example, if you feel like you never have enough money, you may be holding onto excess weight to ensure your survival through tough times or to make you feel less like you have nothing.)

Another set-up statement could be: "Even though I'm overweight and I hate having all this excess fat on my body, I accept that this is how I feel about it and I completely love and forgive myself anyway."

If you have a problem saying that you completely love and forgive yourself, then you can reframe it by saying something like "I choose to love and forgive myself" or "I am open to the possibility of loving and forgiving myself".

## 4. The Sequence:

This is the bit that stimulates and balances the body's energy pathways. We tap around the face and body, tapping with two or three fingers on the end points of the primary meridians
While using our reminder phrase from the set-up statement and any other details that seem relevant – the more specific you can be, the more powerful the technique:

- Top of the Head (TH)
- Beginning of the Eyebrow (EB)
- Side of the Eye (SE)
- Under the Eye (UE)
- Under the Nose (UN)
- Chin Point (CH)
- Beginning of the Collarbone (CB)
- Under the Arm (UA)

The Reminder Phrase is quite simple as you need only identify the issue with some brief wording. Depending on your issue, you might say the following at each tapping point...

*"This throbbing pain"*
*"My fat belly and huge thighs"*
*"Abandoned by my father"*
*"This stuttering in public"*

There are two points to make here – it doesn't matter which hand you use to tap and it doesn't matter which side you tap on, you can tap on either or both.

**5. Test the Intensity Again:**
Finally, you establish an 'after' level of the issue's intensity by rating it on a scale from zero to 10. So, if your issue is a 2 it's not so strong but if it's a 9 or 10 it's as strong as it can be. Don't stress too much about this, just use your intuition and gut feeling. The reason for giving it a score or a number at the start is so that you have something to measure after a few rounds of tapping. You'll be able to see if your feelings get stronger or if they stay the same or lose their intensity. Ideally, the number will get to zero but you may find that it actually goes up initially as you focus on the feelings and thereby increase their intensity as you dive deeper into these emotions. That's all good! You've got to go into them in order to process and release them. Keep tapping until the number starts falling. Keep repeating the tapping process until you get to zero or you plateau at some level.
When you get to a 2 or 3 on the zero to 10 scale, you can try bringing in positive statements, for example, staying with the theme of weight you could say:

*"I choose to love and appreciate my body for a change"*
*"It's time to stop beating myself up about my weight and start recognizing the incredible organism that my body is"*
*"I love and appreciate everything my incredible body does for me"*
*"I am beautiful"*

What I like to do after each round of tapping is cross my hands over my heart, close my eyes and take a deep breath then say the word *'transform'*. I then visualise every cell of my body integrating this new positive belief system and vibrating at this new frequency

Those are the basics in a nutshell. Shall we get on with some really transformational work? Yes, let's do it...

# 3 DEFUSE THE SELF-BLAME

The first thing to address before getting into some of your deeper beliefs and programmes that relate to your weight is to stop the pointless self-judgment, self-blame and criticism for not having the body of your dreams. As well, it's time to play with the idea that counting calories and endless dieting is not working and will never work. If you can kick the dieting habit completely, fantastic! But if you're not ready for that, just allow your brain to consider the notion that dieting is a waste of time.

Beating yourself up for being overweight is never, ever going to get you thinner. You cannot shame yourself slim and happy. You cannot hate yourself slim and happy. You cannot bully, criticize, judge or berate yourself thin. On the contrary, this relentless internal dialogue of self abuse is the perfect way to make sure the excess weight never goes away.
So to kick off this whole new road you're now walking down, begin with the following script for defusing all that old, negative self blame.

Say the set-up statement three times while tapping on the karate chop point of either hand:

*1. Even though, I hate being overweight and it's hard to believe that just dieting harder isn't the answer, and I don't know if I can stop judging myself, I completely love, forgive and accept myself.*

*2. Even though, I've been dieting for so long now that I don't know how not to diet, I honour, love and accept myself anyway.*

*3. Even though I'm scared to even think about not dieting, I don't know how to function outside of the diet mentality, I accept that I feel like this and I love myself anyway.*

Take a deep breath and start tapping around the eight meridian points on the body...

EB: *I don't know how to stop dieting*
SE: *I don't know how to stop hating myself for being overweight*
UE: *If I stop dieting, I'm afraid I'll pack on even more fat*
UN: *It's not safe to stop dieting*
CH: *I don't know how to love myself while I have this weight*
CB: *If I don't beat myself up about my weight, how will it ever shift?*
UN: *No, it's not safe to stop dieting*
TH: *I need to keep driving myself with self-criticism or I'll never lose weight...*
EB: *I don't know how to loathing my body*
SE: *I don't know how to stop feeling like a failure for all this weight*
UE: *How can I possibly love myself when I look like this?*
UN: *How can I accept myself when I look like this?*
CH: *No, it's impossible!*
CB: *If I accept myself like this, I'm afraid I'll stay like this*
UN: *No, it's better if I keep judging and criticising myself*

TH: *That way I'll be motivated to stick to my diet and lose weight*
EB: *By saying I accept myself at this weight*
SE: *Surely I'm saying it's ok to be this overweight?*
UE: *And it's not ok! I can't accept myself looking like this!*
UN: *How can I accept myself when I look like this?*
CH: *I refuse to accept all this excess fat – I hate it!*
CB: *I must keep up the pressure on myself to lose weight*
UN: *I wonder why it never seems to work though*
TH: *I wonder why all these years of self-criticism and dieting haven't worked*
EB: *I might lose a bit of weight but it always come back*
SE: *And I always think that's my fault*
UE: *But what if I've just been going about this the wrong way?*
UN: *What if I've been given wrong information?*
CH: *What if everything I've been told about calories in and calories out is just flawed and misleading information*
CB: *What if dieting and self-loathing is not the answer*
UA: *What if I could let that all go now*
TH: *And find a kinder, easier way to live my life?*

Keep tapping around the body until you've run out of all the fears you have about stopping dieting and stopping self criticism and you feel ready to consider some new ways of thinking, then continue tapping...

EB: *Maybe I could have a new relationship with food*
SE: *Maybe dieting has failed me*
UE: *I've been committed to dieting but it hasn't worked*
UN: *Is it possible that dieting is the problem?*
CH: *What if I could love myself exactly as I am?*
CB: *What if I don't need to hate my belly/thighs/arms...*
UA: *What if my body knows how to heal? If I just got out of the way?*

TH: *What if all the shame and self blame just makes things worse?*
EB: *I know that my body is actually amazing*
SE: *My body works tirelessly to keep me alive and well yet all I do is criticise my beautiful body*
UE: *Maybe, just for today, I can suspend all self-judgment*
UN: *Instead of self-judgment, I'm going to try self-appreciation*
CH: *Maybe I can learn to listen to my body*
CB: *I choose to honour and respect my body*
UA: *I choose to nourish and care for my incredible body*
TH: *I choose to love and appreciate myself*

Continue tapping positive statements around the body until you feel finished. A good sign is when you naturally want to take some big deep breaths or you feel like yawning.

When you're bringing the session to an end, tap on the left side of the fingernails of one hand one by one and say:

*"There's a divine part of me that already knows how to honour, love, nourish and respect my body; that divine part of me is communicating this knowing to the rest of me now; this new knowing is uploaded into every cell of my mind and body now; this process is complete."*

Now, with your eyes closed, cross your hands over your chest, take a deep breath and say *"transform"*.

In your mind's eye, imagine this new knowledge of how to honour, nourish and listen to your body pouring into every cell of your body until your whole being vibrates with this new frequency of self-love. Visualise this happening.

# 4 FIND YOUR BENEFITS

Believe me, I know it's difficult for a hardcore, long-term dieter to accept that there's a part of them that wants all this fat hanging off their frame. But none of us are victims. Whatever you have in your life has a reason for being there, this includes your weight.
The beautiful thing about this way of looking at the world is that if you've created this, you can recreate it. It's a powerful position to be in, the only problem is that we often don't know how we created something and we don't know how to recreate it!
Ultimately, you need to find out how it's serving you, what are the secondary gains, or the pay offs, of this situation?
Be prepared for uncovering some quite screwed up 'benefits' though - remember, your subconscious mind doesn't operate in the same way as your logical conscious mind. For example, people who get sick all the time may have learnt as a child that it's only when they're ill that they get love and attention from their mother or father, thus the subconscious belief is formed 'I must be sick to be loved'.
In fact, I had a client with chronic rheumatoid arthritis who, in the process of unraveling her condition, admitted that it was her "winning card". She said, "no one argues when I play the arthritis card". So part of her healing was learning new ways to define her

boundaries.

For me, I had some very bizarre and often conflicting beliefs and secondary gains around my weight. I used food as both a rebellion against specific people as well as against society as a whole with its rules about how women must look, act and behave.

I also used dieting and weight to bond with my mother - it was the battle we fought together and part of me believed it made us closer. And here's the thing. It did make us closer in a way but it wasn't a healthy way to bond and there are many other more nourishing and loving ways I can be close to my mother without the disempowering closeness of battling weight together.

One of my biggest 'benefits' though was avoiding love relationships because of a belief that 'men abandon me' and 'people who love me, leave me' and 'it's not safe to be happy because people will try to take your happiness away...' I also had beliefs about the weight protecting me from sexual abuse. Yep! I had some issues! And I still have my issues, it's an ongoing process. The key is being able to love and accept yourself right now, as you are, complete with all the emotional scars and baggage that are showing up in your physical body.

So let's start finding some of your limiting beliefs and benefits. I've got an exercise for you to do, you'll need to write things down...

## EXERCISE 1: WHAT'S THE PAY-OFF?

*What would be the worst thing, or the down sides, to losing all your excess weight?*

You may have to really think long and hard about your answers to this question because they may not be immediately obvious - and don't be afraid to write down stuff that your logical head thinks is just silly, e.g., 'God will see me and realise I'm a failure'.

To get you thinking, here are some examples of beliefs and benefits I've come across in my clients and myself...

*"If I'm successful at losing weight, I'll have to be on a diet for the rest of my life to maintain it"*

*"If I lose the weight, I'll have no excuse for not pursuing my dream..."*

*"If I lose weight I'll be happy and I don't deserve to be happy"*

*"If I lose weight and pursue my dream and fail, I can't blame the weight, it'll be all my fault... and I will fail because I'm a failure"*

*"If I lose weight, I'll be giving into all the misogynist cultural and social pressures on women that I resent so much"*

*"If I lose weight, I'll be judged more harshly and I'll attract more jealous criticism"*

*"If I lose weight, I'll be more attractive and might wreck my marriage by going back to my promiscuous ways..."* and so on.

There are thousands of benefits and beliefs around being overweight. Use the rest of this page to write down some of yours... brainstorm with yourself and just write what comes, even if your logical brain thinks your reasons are crazy:

*"The worst thing about losing weight and keeping it off would be...*

# 5 FAT AS PROTECTION

Body fat is used to achieve so many things. When it comes to protecting us, some people use fat to avoid unwanted sexual attention or as a buffer against emotional abuse. They are literally putting on a suit of fat armour. Extra padding for protection.
The subconscious mind detects a threat of some kind and so it instructs the body to uses extra weight as protection. So as far as the body is concerned, this weight is not the problem, it's the solution! So to stop the body-brain using fat in this way, it's not the fat that must be attacked, it's the problem that must be addressed. So, the first question is, what is the perceived problem? If you've done the previous exercise, you'll probably have a list of limiting beliefs or benefits to choose from. Pick the one you'd like to start working with that has to do with how the excess weight protects you, for example, 'being overweight protects me from abuse' or 'this fat puts a buffer between me and that bully'.

Next, go through the following exercises to get a little more information that can be used in the tapping rounds…

**1.  Find the feelings**
Close your eyes, take a few deep breaths, say the belief in your

head and notice where it lives in your body and the emotions that are attached to it, for example, when I say 'being overweight protects me from abuse' I feel it in my belly or solar plexus chakra and it brings up a feeling of being dirty or soiled, and I feel the nine-year-old me come forward and she feels vulnerable.

## 2.  Notice where the weight is

The areas of your body where you are holding extra fat can be a clue as to the purpose it's serving. For example on the rear of the body can mean 'I need to get people off my back; I'm afraid of being attacked from behind'.

If you're a woman and you're holding weight on your belly, it mean 'I regret not having had a baby' or 'I'm losing my children as they grow up and no longer need me' or 'I feel pointless as a woman now that I'm in menopause'. If you're holding weight on your hips and bottom, it could mean something like: 'I want to avoid sexual intimacy' or 'I want to protect my sexual organs'. Some great books for more information on the significance of where we store weight on our body include *Your Body Speaks Your Mind* by Deb Shapiro and *Metaphysical Anatomy* by Evette Rose.

Put your hand on a weight area of particular concern to you, for example your tummy, bottom, arms, thighs etc. Close your eyes, take a couple of deep breaths and ask: 'Why did I choose to put on weight here? What am I holding onto here? What limiting beliefs am I holding in this part of my body? What feelings am I protecting with this weight? What is the emotion here?'

## 3.  Decide on the belief you want to start with

We're going to tap on this first along with the emotions, memories and feelings it brings up. Use your own words but the following Tapping script can be used as a guide. The most important thing is to say whatever feels raw and true and intense. If saying it makes you feel teary or emotional in some way – you've hit a nerve, which is good!

Rate the intensity of this belief from zero to 10 and then say the set-up statement three times while tapping on the karate chop point of either hand:

1.   *Even though part of me believes my weight protects me from abuse, I still completely love and accept myself*

2. *Even though I'm holding onto this excess weight to protect myself from abuse that's made me feel dirty, I honour, love and accept myself anyway*

3. *Even though my body and mind needs this extra weight to feel safe from abuse, and I feel this fear and sadness in my belly, I still profoundly love and accept myself exactly as I am.*

EB: *I'm holding onto sadness and fear in my belly*
SE: *This fat on my belly is protecting me from attack*
UE: *The little child in me is terrified of being abused again*
UN: *The little child in me believes this fat stops me from being abused again and maybe she's right*
CH: *I'd much rather stay fat than be abused*
CB: *So maybe I do need to keep this fat on my body for protection*
UA: *The thought of the abuse makes me feel sick in my stomach*
TH: *It makes me feel dirty and sad*

Take a slow and deep breath.
Keep tapping around the body until you've run out of things to say about your belief and benefit.
Take a moment to rate the intensity of the belief now. Is it down to three or below?

If so and you feel ready to consider some new more positive ways of thinking, then continue tapping...

EB: *What if there are better ways to stay safe now?*
SE: *I'm not a little child anymore*
UE: *That was then but this is now*
UN: *And I'm open to new ways of operating in the world*
CH: *I no longer need the weight to stay safe from abuse*
CB: *I have much better tools now*
UA: *I release this sadness and fear of abuse now*
TH: *I choose to believe I am safe in this world*

Continue tapping positive statements around the body until you feel finished. A good sign is when you naturally want to take some big deep breaths or you feel like yawning.
When you're ready to finish, tap on the left side of each of your fingernails on one hand one by one, saying:

*"There is a divine part of me that already knows how to honour, love, nourish and respect my body; that divine part of me is communicating this knowing to the rest of me now; this new knowing is uploaded into every cell of my mind and body now; this process is complete."*

Now, with your eyes closed, cross your hands over your chest, take a deep breath and say *"transform"*.

In your mind's eye, imagine this new knowledge of how to honour, nourish and listen to your body pouring into every cell of your body until your whole being vibrates with this new frequency of self-love..

# 6 FAT AS LOVE

If you have wonderful memories of eating food with people who love you and who nurtured you then chances are you have a 'fat is love' belief knocking around in your subconscious mind. This is when we store our feelings in the food. As a result, the good feelings and loving memories are also stored in your fat.

Use your own words but the following example can be used as a guide. The most important thing is to say whatever feels raw and true.

Rate the intensity of this belief from zero to 10 and then say the set-up statement three times while tapping on the karate chop point of either hand:

*1. Even though, part of me perceives food and love as the same thing, I forgive myself and I completely love and accept myself*

*2. Even though part of me feels loved and comforted when I eat certain foods, I completely love and accept myself regardless.*

*3. Even though part of me feels loved and nourished when I eat foods that are sweet treats, I accept that these are my feelings and I honour and accept myself.*

EB: *I eat to feel loved*
SE: *Eating certain foods makes me feel soothed and comforted*
UE: *Certain foods bring back happy memories*
UN: *And happy feelings*
CH: *Good times were celebrated with food*
CB: *Food was a treat and a reward*
UA: *I was rewarded with food*
TH: *Now I use food to reward myself*
EB: *Eating comforting foods makes me feel good*
SE: *So I hold onto all this excess love-fat*
UE: *Eating reminds me of being loved*
UN: *Eating reminds me of people I love*
CH: *Eating reminds me of people who love me*
CB: *Eating with loved ones is a celebration*
UA: *A time to relax and enjoy*
TH: *It's no wonder I use food to feel loved*
EB: *Our lives revolve around food and fun times*
SE: *From baking with grandma, to sharing chocolate with friends, and sharing cake with my mum…food is love*
UE: *So it's no surprise that I turn to food when I need cheering up*
UN: *Food is my drug of choice*
CH: *The only problem is that all this food love is making me fat*
CB: *And I really don't love that*
UA: *Because the truth is that food isn't love*
TH: *Food as a poor substitute for genuine love*
EB: *And frankly I deserve better*
SE: *I deserve real love and nourishment*
UE: *Food is not love*
UN: *Love is love*

*CH: All this love-fat is not love*
*CB: Food cannot love me*
*UA: Food does not cherish and value me*
*TH: Comfort foods cannot give me the body and life I want*

Take several deep breaths. If you have anything else you want to 'talk and tap out', continue tapping around the meridian points while saying whatever you intuitively know you need to say; whatever feels true and raw and visceral. Speak whatever your soul calls you to express. When all that is out and you feel ready to instill new supportive beliefs with positive statement, move on to something like the following…

*EB: I'm ready to love myself in a new way*
*SE: I'm ready to love and nourish myself in a healthy way*
*UE: I know how to love myself without misusing food*
*UN: I know how to love myself without abusing food*
*CH: I have better ways to reward myself*
*CB: I no longer need food to feel loved*
*UA: I know that I am loved*
*TH: I know how to love and reward myself without food*
*EB: I am excited to be freed from this old addiction*
*SE: I'm excited about finding new ways to feel loved*
*UE: I am loved*
*UN: I don't need food to feel loved*
*CH: I have my wonderful memories*
*CB: Food is not love*
*UA: I deserve real love*
*TH: I have better ways of treating myself*
*EB: I have more exciting ways to feel good*
*SE: So maybe I can let go of all this excess love-fat*
*UE: Maybe I can shed all this love-fat*
*UN: Because it's not real love*

*CH: Yes, it's reminding me of real love*

*CB: But I can be reminded of real love without the kilos of love-fat*

*UA: So I choose to have a new relationship with food*

*TH: I choose to release this love-fat*

*EB: I don't need this love-fat*

*SE: I choose to fully engage with life*

*UE: I choose to know and feel true love*

*UN: I love myself too much to punish my body with food*

*CH: I love my body too much to punish it with food*

*CB: I choose to honour my body and myself*

*UA: And I make the command now to sever all connections that my brain makes between food and love*

*TH: I command now that my subconscious mind cancels the belief that food is love*

*EB: I command now that my subconscious mind cancels the belief that love and food are interchangeable*

*SE: I command that a new belief is programmed into my subconscious mind*

*UE: I command to know what it feels like and how to live my life without substituting food for love*

*UN: I command to know what it feels like and how to live my life without holding onto excess fat as a reminder of love*

*CH: I know what it feels like and how to live my life without believing that food is love*

*CB: I choose real love*

*UA: I choose to love and honour myself*

*TH: Real love is my birthright*

Close your eyes, cross the hands over your heart, and take three deep breaths, then say 'transform'.

In your mind's eye, imagine this new knowledge of how to honour, nourish and listen to your body pouring into every cell of your body until your whole being vibrates with this new frequency of self-love. Witness this happening.

# 7 FAT AS AN EXCUSE

Excess weight is a great excuse for putting life on hold. I did it for decades. Sometimes it's big things and other times it's small things. For example, you might say to yourself, 'I'll start dating once I've lost weight', 'I'll join that yoga class when I've lost weight', 'I'll look for a new job when I lose weight', 'I'll reward myself to that motorcycle tour of South America when I've lost weight'.

Or you might think to yourself, 'I'll buy new underwear when I've lost weight', 'I'll get a manicure and my hair cut when I've lost weight'. There is no end to the things we deny and deprive ourselves of as some kind of carrot and stick method for losing weight. It doesn't work and all it really achieves is reinforcing the belief in your subconscious that you're not good enough as you are; that you don't deserve a fun and satisfying life as the person you are right now.

But that's not all. Many of us also use eating as a distraction and a method of procrastination. Distractions are a way to not face life and to avoid our problems but at the same time keeping ourselves busy.

Eating isn't the only pastime we humans use to distract ourselves. We also use movies, TV shows, magazines, gambling, social media, gossip, video games, internet surfing, football, collecting teddy bears, obsessive cleaning, … and so on. Why do we do this? We distract ourselves under the premise of 'if I'm not looking at the problems, the problems will go away'. A similar approach is sticking one's fingers into one's ears and singing 'la la la la la…'

However when we continually duck and dive our way through life instead of facing our challenges, we are telling ourselves that we incapable and cowardly. So while they may seem like innocent pastimes, buying into these distractions can be extremely damaging and disempowering. In the case of using food as a distraction, the issue is broader. As well as the burden that the excess weight places on your frame and joints as a result of this distraction eating, the effect of eating as a distraction is that we stuff down our emotions instead of feeling and processing them. We silence our soul and spirit with food and the unresolved emotional baggage manifests as physical baggage that we carry with us every moment of every day. Wouldn't you like to let go of all that?

The following tapping script can be used as a guide but if you feel inclined, change the words to suit your own situation. Speak whatever comes to mind; whatever feelings and thoughts demand to be finally spoken. The most important thing is to say whatever feels raw and true.

Rate the intensity of this belief from zero to 10 and then say the set-up statement three times while tapping on the karate chop point of either hand:

*1. Even though I use food and eating to distract myself, I honour and love myself anyway*

*2. Even though, I eat to distract myself from facing life, I forgive myself and respect how I feel*

*3. Even though, I avoid facing life by distracting myself with food, I completely love, honour and accept myself anyway*

*EB: I distract myself with food*
*SE: I eat to distract myself from life*
*UE: I avoid life by eating*
*CH: I use food as a distraction*
*CB: I use food as a distraction*
*UA: I eat to distract myself*
*TH: I eat to avoid life*
*EB: I eat to avoid my feelings*
*SE: I eat to suppress my feelings and thoughts about my life*
*UE: All these things I want to be distracted from*
*CH: I don't want to face all these things*
*CB: It's painful to face up to all these things*
*UA: I feel overwhelmed*
*TH: All the worries and doubts and stress consume me*
*EB: I don't want to face all that! Who would?!*
*SE: So instead I choose to consume*
*UE: Eating is a life silencer*
*CH: I don't want to feel and I don't want to think*
*CB: I need a distraction*
*UA: So I use food and drink*
*TH: It's a wonderful distraction*
*EB: But it comes with some unwanted side effects*
*SE: All this fat on my body*

*UE: This excess fat is my avoidance made manifest*
*CH: It's the physical result of distracting myself with food*
*CB: Maybe distracting myself is causing more pain than it's avoiding*
*UA: Distracting myself with food is damaging my health*
*TH: Distracting myself with food is disempowering*
*EB: Distracting myself with food is hurting me*
*SE: Distracting myself with food is keeping me stuck*
*UE: I'm ready to find out what I'm distracting myself from*
*CH: I'm ready to face what I've been avoiding with food*
*CB: I'm ready to change my distraction habits*
*UA: I'm ready to feel what I've been afraid to feel*
*TH: I'm ready to stop distracting myself with food*

With your eyes closed, take three deep breaths in through the nose and out through the mouth. Let this new information start decoding the old information in your DNA. See as your old patterns and habits start to loosen and release. If any other memories or feelings have surfaced, tap on them. Then, when you feel ready, continue on to the next section of tapping.

*EB: Maybe I no longer need to distract myself with food*
*SE: Maybe it's time to face my feelings*
*UE: Maybe it's time to feel and heal*
*UN: Maybe that won't be so bad!*
*CH: Maybe being fully present with how I feel isn't so hard*
*CB: All these things I've been avoiding*
*UA: All the emotions I've been avoiding*
*TH: Maybe there's nothing I can't deal with*
*EB: I choose to recognize when I'm distracting myself with food*
*SE: I make different choices now*
*UE: Maybe I'm stronger than I realise*
*UN: Maybe I'm more resourceful and capable than I realise*

*CH: I don't need to avoid life by eating*
*CB: I want to live my life to the fullest*
*UA: I want to feel love and joy and happiness*
*TH: I might not get it right all the time*
*EB: But I won't beat myself up*
*SE: I'll let myself transform these habits at my own pace*
*UE: I'll notice when I want to distract myself with eating*
*UN: And I'll take the time to look at what I'm avoiding*
*CH: I choose to live life fully*
*CB: I choose to live life fearlessly*
*UA: I choose to feel my feelings*
*TH: I choose to welcome life*
*EB: I choose to honour my feelings in healthier ways*
*SE: I choose to let self-sabotaging habits fall away*
*UE: I make new choices*
*UN: I notice when I'm distracting myself*
*CH: And I gently and lovingly make different choices*
*CB: I honour my body and its wellness*
*UA: I love myself unconditionally.*
*TH: And so it is*

With the eyes closed, cross your hands over your chest, take three deep breaths and say 'transform'.

Watch as every cell of your body absorbs and reflects this new information.

Watch your cells release the old patterns and witness the new choices being encoded into your DNA.

Mindfully open your eyes onto a whole new world in which you no longer use food as a distraction or for procrastination. A world in which you no longer use your excess body fat as an excuse.

# 8 FAT AS SAFETY

Hiding within a soft cocoon of fat can feel like a nice, cosy and safe place to be.

People cushion themselves in layers of excess weight to stay safer in so many ways. For example, some people gain weight when they get married as a way to avoid being unfaithful, other people use weight to feel that they're not so easy to push around – they literally feel more stable and solid with this extra weight.

I had a client who was subconsciously holding onto a considerable amount of excess weight because he was a university lecturer whose job was to teach in large lecture halls that seated up to 300 people. So as not to feel insignificant and unseen in such a large space, he made himself bigger.

Similarly, for people who grew up believing that being overweight was a family trait and in order to really feel like they belonged in their family they must be overweight, then holding onto excess fat allows them to feel like a loved and valued member of the family.

If you have some beliefs and benefits around using fat as a way to keep yourself safe, try using this script as a basis for tapping around your specific issues.

As before, use your own words whenever you feel inclined and the most important thing is to say whatever feels raw and true.

Rate the intensity of this belief from zero to 10 and then say the set-up statement three times while tapping on the karate chop point of either hand:

*1. Even though I've been keeping myself overweight to hold myself back in life, I choose to love and accept myself.*

*2. Even though, I use excess weight to dim my light and hold myself back in life in order to stay safe, I love, honour and accept myself completely.*

*3. Even though, all this excess weight holds me back in life and that keeps me safe, I still choose to love and respect myself*

*EB: I stay overweight to hold myself back in life*
*SE: It's not safe to stand out*
*UE: It's not safe to shine and draw attention to myself*
*UN: Standing out attracts hatred, jealousy, judgment, and criticism*
*CH: It's not safe to shine my light too brightly*
*CB: It's safer to dim my light*
*UA: It's safer to dull my shine*
*TH: If I'm too successful, people will hate me*
*EB: When I stood out in the past I was judged*
*SE: When I shone my light in the past, I was hated*
*UE: So it's safer to hold myself back in life*
*UN: It's safer to dim my light*
*CH: It's safer to dull my shine*
*CB: Extra weight is a perfect way to hold myself back*
*UA: Excess fat is a great way to dim my light*
*TH: Excess fat is how I dull my shine*
*EB: It's safer that way*

*SE: No one likes a show off*
*UE: Attracting attention attracts hatred*
*UN: No one likes a show off*
*CH: Keeping myself overweight means avoiding jealousy*
*CB: Keeping myself overweight means not being seen*
*UA: Keeping myself overweight means I'm in the shadows*
*TH: Being overweight dims my light*

Take several deep breaths and do any more tapping on anything else that's come up, for example, a specific memory before the age of eight when you received negative feedback when you attracted attention. Perhaps you got criticized when you played the lead in the school play, perhaps the others in your dance class ganged up on you when you were chosen as the main dancer, perhaps your mother told you to stop showing off when you were the centre of attention at your birthday party… or whatever. When you feel finished with tapping on the negatives, move to the next part…

*EB: Maybe it's safe now to shine my light*
*SE: Maybe I can shine my light and receive accolades and appreciation*
*UE: Maybe I can stand out without attracting hatred*
*UN: Maybe there's a big difference between shining my light and showing off*
*CH: And I know what that difference is*
*CB: Maybe I can fully use all my gifts and talents*
*UA: In fact, it's insulting to God if I don't fully use all my gifts and talents*
*TH: I dishonour myself and God when I dim my light*
*EB: I honour God and myself when I shine my light as brightly as possible*
*SE: And it's fun to shine!*

*UE: It's safe to shine!*
*UN: Maybe I can be impervious to haters*
*CH: The world needs more light*
*CB: The world needs my light*
*UA: The world needs me to shine as brightly as I'm able to*
*TH: So no more holding myself back*
*EB: No more dimming my light with excess weight*
*SE: I choose to shed the weight and shine my light*
*UE: I know it's possible and it's safe to stand out*
*UN: I choose to be seen*
*CH: I choose to attract positive attention*
*CB: I choose to shine brightly*
*UA: I choose to step into the spotlight*
*TH: It's safe to shed this weight and shine my light brightly*

Side of hand: *I now release any and all resistance to releasing the need to hold onto the excess fat on my body. I release any and all resistance I have anywhere in the universe, anywhere in me, anywhere in my thinking, anywhere in my history, anywhere in my experience, anywhere in my energy field to releasing excess body fat effortlessly, easily, in a quick and healthy way.*

Take three deep breaths, cross your hands over your chest and with your eyes closed, say '*transform*'. Feel your heart beating beneath your hands and mindfully open your eyes on a new world in which you no longer resist the release of excess body fat.

# 9 FAT AS SURVIVAL

If someone has financial or job worries, or if their ancestors experienced famine, this can result in holding onto excess weight. Our ancestors' fears of famine and starvation can be passed down in our DNA thus explaining our primal fear of famine even though we may be in an environment where food is abundant. Ironically, it is dieting that can trigger the genetic patterning of famine fear and set in motion the body-brain's tools for protecting you against famine.
I believe that everyone who's spent years on a diet has triggered their famine response to kick in on an epic scale. That's what low calorie dieting achieves. It puts your body into emergency mode and it can stay there for years and years – constantly doing everything it can to fight the loss of excess fat.

Try this Tapping Script for Ancestral Famine. Start by saying the set-up statement three times, taking a deep breath after each one.

*1. Even though, part of me is clinging onto extra body fat for fear of famine and starvation, I still completely love and accept myself*

*2. Even though, part of me is scared that there's not going to be enough so I need to save for a rainy day, I accept my feelings and love myself anyway*

*3. Even though, part of me doesn't believe that I'll always have enough, I still profoundly love and accept myself*


*EB: Somewhere inside me there is a deep fear of famine and lack*
*SE: This deep terror of starving*
*UE: Somewhere in my DNA, I'm terrified of famine and starvation*
*UN: Famine and starvation*
*CH: I'm terrified of starving to death*
*CB: Because it's happened before*
*UA: It's happened to me in past lives*
*TH: And it's happened to my ancestors*
*EB: The horror of famine can happen*
*SE: So part of me wants to be prepared for that*
*UE: I need to stockpile*
*UN: I need to make sure I've got reserves in*
*CH: I need to be ready for an emergency*
*CB: This extra weight will keep me alive in a famine*
*UA: This extra weight will protect me from starvation*
*TH: I feel safer when I have this extra weight with me*
*EB: I might die without this extra weight*
*SE: I know that can happen, it happens all the time*
*UE: People starve to death all over the world*
*UN: You never know what the future holds*
*CH: So it's safer if I store away as much as I can in case of disaster*
*CB: I feel protected and safer when I'm carrying extra weight*
*UA: Although there are many downsides to holding onto this extra weight as well*
*TH: Carrying all this extra fat is tough on my body*

*EB: This extra weight hurts my joints and my organs*
*SE: My body has to work a lot harder with all this extra weight*
*UE: It might even cause me to die a lot sooner than I would
without it*
*UN: That's probably more likely to happen than famine*
*CH: So it would be great if I didn't need to load my body with
extra fat in case of an emergency*
*UA: But what else can I do to survive famine?*
*TH: What if there was another way though?*
*EB: What if I other options for surviving famine*
*SE: What if I could survive famine without carrying all this extra
weight?*
*UE: And maybe my amazing body already has built in tools for
tackling periods of famine?*
*UN: Maybe all this extra weight just makes my body's job harder*
*CH: Maybe my body already knows how to survive famine…*
*CB: …without me holding so much extra fat*
*UA: It has a built in famine response that adjusts my body's
chemistry*
*TH: It has already allowed for extra energy in emergency
situations*
*EB: It doesn't need or want the many extra kilograms that I've
packed on*
*SE: That's like jumping into a lifeboat with so many suitcases that
the lifeboat sinks*
*UE: So maybe this is the wrong way to go about preparing for
famine*
*UN: Maybe I do have some past experience of famine*
*CH: That doesn't mean it will happen again in this life*
*CB: I live in an abundant universe*
*UA: I live on an abundant planet that supports all living things*
*TH: My body is an exquisite, ever-evolving and intelligent
organism*

*EB: My body is connected to a creative force that's much wiser than my conscious mind*
*SE: I trust my body's wisdom in caring for me*
*UE: I trust that my body knows best how to look after itself*
*UN: I trust that my body has a vast array of tools to be used for surviving and thriving*
*CH: So maybe I can let this extra body fat go now*
*CB: Maybe I don't need to be locked into the fear of famine*
*UA: If famine ever does come, I'll deal with it then*
*TH: There's no need to be ever-ready for a famine that may never occur*
*EB: It's like living life through the cross hairs of a loaded gun*
*SE: It's time to stop living from a place of fear*
*UE: It's time to start living from a place of love and safety*
*UN: I know what it feels like to always have plenty*
*CH: I know what it feels like to be abundant*
*CB: I know what it feels like to be prosperous*
*UA: I let go of the fear now*
*TH: I let go of the fat now*
*EB: I release the fear and the fat now*
*SE: I release all fear of famine from every cell of my body now*
*UE: There is a part of me that already knows how to live without this fear of famine*
*UN: That part of me is informing the rest of me now*
*CH: This new information is pouring like white light into every cell of my physical and etheric bodies now*
*CB: My mind, body and spirit are now sparkling with the light of this new information*
*UA: I release all fear of famine from every cell of my body now*
*TH: And so it is*

Close your eyes, cross your arms over your heart, say 'transform' and take three deeps breaths.

# 10 LOVE LETTER TO MY BODY

Well done you amazing, brilliant, gorgeous creature, you made it!
You're here, at the end of this book.
I hope you're a brighter, emotionally lighter being now than you
were when you started this transformation process. I hope you've
had a shift of some kind no matter how small. I hope you've had a
revelation, an epiphany, an 'aha' moment or a realization about
yourself, your life, your power and your potential.
Because you really are amazing and divine. And the body you
navigate and experience this physical 3D world in is also amazing
and divine.
Maybe this marks the beginning of a new path for you.
Regardless of where you are at on your path, I wish you every
success in breaking the old habits that were keeping you fat and
unhappy.
I wish you every success in seeing yourself in a whole new light
and knowing that it all starts and ends with self-love.
As I said at the start, you cannot hate yourself thin. You cannot
shame, guilt, or berate yourself thin. It works the other way
around. Once you love yourself enough, your body will no longer
reflect your emotional baggage as excess weight. So with that in
mind, here is a final tapping script. I recommend you do this as

often as you can, maybe try going through this script every morning for a week… or longer if you can.

*1. Even though my body carries more fat on it than I think is desirable, I still completely love and accept myself*

*2. Even though I'm carrying more fat on my body than I believe is desirable and I would like to release some of this excess fat, I know that my body has good reasons for keeping this weight and I completely love and accept myself regardless.*

*3. Even though my body is holding more fat that I would like and I feel bad about feeling bad about myself, I accept that these are my feelings and I honour how I feel.*

*EB: My dearest body*
*SE: I've directed a lot of hate at you over the years*
*UE: I've criticized you*
*UN: I've judged you*
*CH: I've deprived you*
*CB: I've been ashamed of you*
*UA: I've punished you*
*TH: I've abused you*
*EB: I've rejected you*
*SE: I've hated you*
*UE: I've told you that there was something wrong with you*
*UN: I've compared you unfavourably with other bodies*
*CH: Telling you you're not as good as them*
*CB: I haven't appreciated you*
*UA: I've taken you for granted*
*TH: I haven't looked after you properly*
*EB: I've filled you with toxins and pollutants and chemicals*
*SE: I've over stuffed you with unnatural foods*

*UE: I've overloaded you, tripling your workload in order to keep me healthy*
*UN: And then I've still found fault with you*
*CH: I've forgotten what an incredible gift you are*
*CB: I've forgotten that you are a walking miracle*
*UA: I've forgotten that just one cell of you is more brilliant and more intelligent than all the best computers on earth put together*
*TH: I've failed to nurture you properly*
*EB: I've failed to take proper care of you*
*SE: I've failed to give you enough quality food, water, air and sleep*
*UE: And yet still you work for me tirelessly, relentlessly and thanklessly*
*UN: Dearest body, please forgive me*
*CH: Forgive me for the love I've denied you*
*CB: Forgive me for the acceptance I've denied you*
*UA: Forgive me for insulting and rejecting you*
*TH: I'm ready to change my ways*

Take three deep breaths and if you feel ready, continue tapping…

*EB: Dearest body, please forgive me*
*SE: I know that every single thing you do is for my benefit*
*UE: I know you have some really good reasons for holding onto this excess body fat*
*UN: I know that you believe I need this extra fat*
*CH: And as long as you believe I need this fat*
*CB: You will fight to keep it where it is*
*UA: And you're doing this because you love me*
*TH: Maybe this fat makes us feel safer against the threat of famine*
*EB: Maybe this fat makes us feel bigger and stronger when facing the world*

*SE: Maybe this fat is our emotional armour*
*UE: Maybe this fat is a substitute for love and affection*
*UN: Maybe this fat keeps unwanted sexual attention at bay*
*CH: Maybe this fat is storing all the emotions and feelings that I dare not express*
*CB: Maybe this fat is keeping heavy metals in quarantine where they can't hurt my organs and brain*
*UA: Maybe this fat is filling an emotional hole within me*
*TH: Maybe this fat gives me a great excuse for not living life fully*
*EB: Maybe this fat is about rebelling against a world that refuses to approve of me*
*SE: Maybe this fat is about something else completely*
*UE: Dearest body, I know you have good reasons for keeping this fat*
*UN: And if you want to keep all this fat, I will no longer fight you*
*CH: I will attempt to understand your good reasons*
*CB: And maybe we can change some of the reasons*
*UA: So maybe you won't feel like there are benefits to keeping the fat anymore*
*TH: But there is no hurry*
*EB: I'm going to start loving you exactly as you are*
*SE: Please be patient with me though*
*UE: I need to change some life-long and deeply engrained patterns*
*UN: Patterns of self-criticism and self-judgment*
*CH: So I may not always be consistent*
*CB: But I will now be aware of when I am not being kind to you*
*UA: And I will change that*
*TH: Dearest body, thank you so much for everything you do to keep me safe and well in this world*
*EB: Thank you for my heart that has pumped about 100,000 times every day since I was born*
*SE: Thank you for the lungs that keep oxygen and prana flowing*

*through my body*
*UE: Thank you for my liver, kidneys, and pancreas*
*UN: Thank you for my skin*
*CH: Thank you for the feet and legs that attach me to this earth and move me wherever I want to go*
*UA: Thank you for my incredible hands that never stop working, creating, expressing*
*TH: Thank you for my bones that give me support and structure*
*EB: Thank you for my eyes, my ears, my nose*
*SE: Thank you for my throat and neck*
*UE: Thank you for my reproductive organs and genitals*
*UN: Thank you for my stomach and intestines and digestive system*
*CH: Thank you for my amazing brain*
*CB: This brain that filters two billion units of information per second…*
*UA: …deciding what I need to notice and what I don't*
*TH: I know there is so much more to my beautiful body than all this…*
*EB: Thank you for every last molecule that forms this incredible vessel*
*SE: This incredible vessel for my soul*
*UE: This miraculous body that enables my soul to experience this 3D world*
*UN: I know I am blessed to have this body*
*CH: Body, I love you*
*CB: Body, thank you, I love you*
*UA: Body, thank you, I love you*
*TH: I love you my beautiful, incredible body*

Close your eyes, cross the hands over your heart, and take three deep breaths, then say '*transform*'.

ABOUT THE AUTHOR

Tamara Pitelen was born in New Zealand to parents who migrated there from the north of England in the 1960s on the £10 boats. Since then, she's lived in Japan, HongKong, Australia, and Dubai but the place she currently calls home is the beautiful city of Bath, where she lives with her husband Adrian, their cat Jake, and an ever-changing number of rescue hens.

As well as having held a 'day job' in print and online media for more than two decades, Tamara is also a certified yoga teacher, a practitioner of EFT Tapping and ThetaHealing. She is passionate about alternative healthcare, energy healing, and spirituality. Tamara has written an Amazon bestselling book about cycling around Ireland; she trained as a yoga teacher and a Reiki practitioner on the banks of the Ganges in Rishikesh, India, and did a stint in stand-up comedy in Australia.

www.tamarapitelen.com

www.ingramcontent.com/pod-product-compliance
Lightning Source LLC
Chambersburg PA
CBHW071238240726
48654CB00009B/1112